Pegan Diet Recipes

Recipes

Tasty Recipes Combining Paleo and Vegan Diets for
Healthy Weight Loss, Longevity and Performance

Ashley Cohan

work can be in any fashion deemed liable for any hardship or damages that may befall them after undertaking information described herein.

Additionally, the information in the following pages is intended only for informational purposes and should thus be thought of as universal. As befitting its nature, it is presented without assurance regarding its prolonged validity or interim quality. Trademarks that are mentioned are done without written consent and can in no way be considered an endorsement from the trademark holder.

TABLE OF CONTENTS

INTRODUCTION

The Pegan diet is a plant based eating style that incorporates concepts of the paleo diet and the vegan diet. The idea is to cut back on the processed stuff as followers of the diet eat vegetables, fruits, nuts, seeds, meat, fish, and eggs and avoid dairy, grains, sugar, and processed foods. The pegan diet encourages good health by reducing inflammation and controlling blood sugar.

The Pegan Diet was created where 60% of your food is made up of carbs and they allow for more green vegetables than some other diets. The Pegan Diet also allows you to consume beans that have a variety of different nutrients including fiber and protein. The Pegan Diet is based on unrefined healthy fat as well as lean protein which are both important factors when it comes to heart health.

The Pegan Diet is similar to the Paleo Diet in that it does not allow refined carbs, processed foods, or dairy products. It is also similar to the Ketogenic Diet in that it does not allow gluten or added sugars. The Pegan Diet is different from both of these diets because it allows for higher carbohydrate intake than either.

Pagans can eat both animal and plant proteins. If a vegetarian means to follow the Pegan diet, it would be very doable! Vegetarian sources of protein include black beans, pinto beans, lentils, edamame, chickpeas, quinoa, nuts, seeds, and more. Many individuals overeat protein while under-eating fresh fruits and vegetables.

The vegan and the Paleo diet reduce the chances of certain diseases. Both of them!

The Pegan diet promises optimal health by reducing inflammation and balancing blood sugar and besides, the Pegan diet has many health benefits, including weight loss, increased energy levels, and reduced risk of diseases such as diabetes, heart disease, obesity, and cancer.

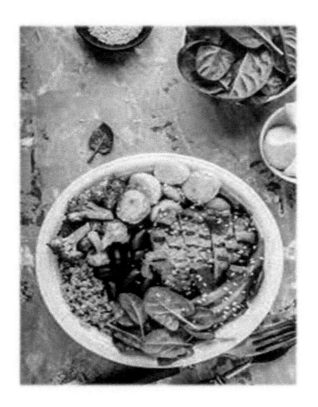

PEGAN RECIPES

Easy Homemade Cashew "Yogurt"

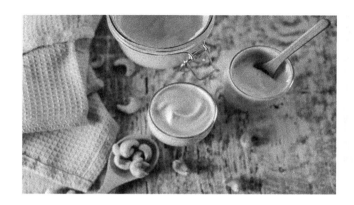

Time required:
30 minutes

Servings: 04

INGREDIENTS

2 cups of cashews, soaked 3 hours or (ideally) overnight

1 teaspoon of psyllium husks + 1/2 cup of filtered water

1 ripe banana

1 teaspoon of vanilla

1 tablespoon of coconut oil

a pinch of sea salt

2 tablespoons of lemon juice about 1/2+ filtered water

To Make A Parfait:

about 1 cup of fresh or frozen berries, such as blueberries,

STEPS FOR COOKING

1. In a small bowl, mix the psyllium husks with water and set aside to allow it to thicken.

2. Drain the soaked cashews, and place them into a high-powered blender, or a food processor. Add the banana, vanilla, coconut oil, salt, and lemon juice. While the blender or food processor is running continuously, add the water in a slow stream. You might need a little more than a 1/2 cup. Add additional water a tablespoon at a time, until the mixture runs smooth, but is still thick and creamy.

3. Transfer the yogurt to a bowl, and stir in the thickened psyllium husks. Place in the fridge for 30 minutes, and then your yogurt is ready to enjoy.

4. If you want to make a parfait, layer your parfait ingredients alternating

raspberries, or blackberries

about 1/2 cup of your favorite granola

additional add ins: bee pollen, chia seeds, hemp seeds

with layers of yogurt. I like to do this in small mason jars and store them (with a tight lid) in the fridge. These will keep for a couple of days in an air-tight container in the fridge.

FROSTED LEMONADE

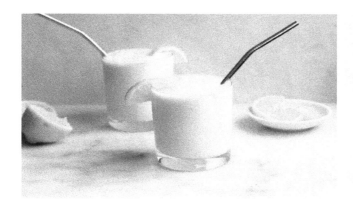

Time required:
10 minutes

Servings: 01

INGREDIENTS

1/2 cup lemon juice or juice of 2 lemons

2/3 cup unsweetened almond milk

2 tablespoons collagen

1/2 teaspoon Now Brand Stevia Extract

2 pinches Himalayan salt or mineral salt

1 teaspoon vanilla extract

1/2 teaspoon glucomannan

3 cups ice cubes (around one full ice tray)

STEPS FOR COOKING

1. Put lemon juice, almond milk, collagen, stevia, salt, and vanilla in a blender. Turn on low for just a few seconds to mix. While blender is on low, slowly add in glucomannan.

2. Blend on low for 30 seconds and turn off. Add in ice cubes and blend on high until ice cubes have been completely blended.

APPLE AND CINNAMON OATMEAL

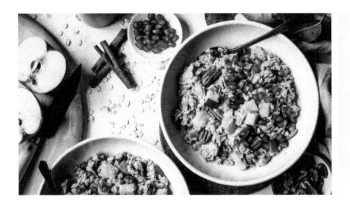

Time required:
20 minutes

Servings: 04

INGREDIENTS

1/4 cups apple cider

1 apple, peeled, cored, and chopped

2/3 cup rolled oats

1 teaspoon ground cinnamon

1 tablespoon pure maple syrup

STEPS FOR COOKING

1. Take the apple cider to a boil over medium-high heat, then stir in the apple, oats, and cinnamon.

2. Bring the cereal to a boil and turn down the heat to low. Simmer until the oatmeal thickens, then spoon into two bowls and sweeten with maple syrup, if using. Serve hot.

ORANGE FRENCH TOAST

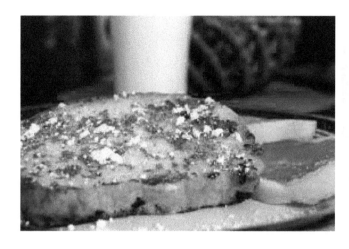

Time required:
20 minutes

Servings: 04

3 very ripe bananas

1 cup unsweetened nondairy milk

Zest and juice of 1 orange

1 teaspoon ground cinnamon

1/4 teaspoon grated nutmeg

4 slices French bread

1 tablespoon coconut oil

1. Blend the bananas, almond milk, orange juice and zest, cinnamon, and nutmeg and blend until smooth. Dip the bread in the mixture for 5 minutes on each side.

2. While the bread soaks, heat a griddle or sauté pan over medium-high heat and melt the coconut oil in the pan and swirl to coat. Cook the bread slices until golden brown on both sides, about 5 minutes each. Serve immediately.

SPICED ORANGE BREAKFAST COUSCOUS

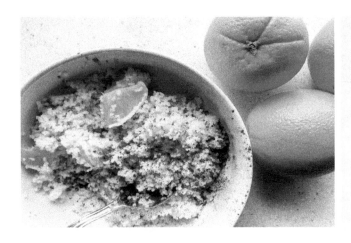

Time required:
20 minutes

Servings: 04

INGREDIENTS

3 cups orange juice

1.1/2 cups couscous

1 teaspoon ground cinnamon

1/4 teaspoon ground cloves

1/2 cup dried fruit

1/2 cup chopped almonds

STEPS FOR COOKING

1. Take the orange juice to a boil. Add the couscous, cinnamon, and cloves, then remove from heat. Shield the pan and allow sitting until the couscous softens.

2. Fluff the couscous and stir in the dried fruit and nuts. Serve immediately. Pecans and syrup. Serve hot.

Pumpkin Pancakes

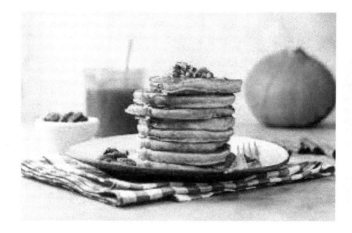

Time required:
20 minutes

Servings: 04

INGREDIENTS

2 cups unsweetened almond milk

1 teaspoon apple cider vinegar

2.1/2 cups whole-wheat flour

2 tablespoons baking powder

1/2 teaspoon baking soda

1 teaspoon sea salt

1 teaspoon pumpkin pie

1/2 cup canned pumpkin purée

1 cup water

1 tablespoon coconut oil

STEPS FOR COOKING

1. Dip together the flour, baking powder, baking soda, salt, and pumpkin pie spice.

2. In another large bowl, combine the almond milk mixture, pumpkin purée, and water, whisking to mix well.

3. Add the wet ingredients to the dry ingredients and fold together until the dry ingredients are just moistened. You will still have a few streaks of flour in the bowl.

4. In a nonstick pan or griddle over medium-high heat, melt the coconut oil and swirl to coat. Pour the batter into the pan 1/4 cup at a time and cook until the pancakes are browned, about 5 minutes per side. Serve immediately.

SMOOTHIE BREAKFAST BOWL

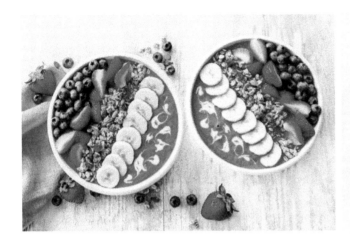

Time required:
30 minutes

Servings: 04

INGREDIENTS

4 bananas, peeled

*1 cup dragon fruit
(or other fruit)*

1 cup Baked Granola

2 cups fresh berries

*1/2 cup slivered
almonds*

*4 cups plant-based
milk*

STEPS FOR COOKING

1. Open 4 quart-size, freezer-safe bags, and layer in the following order: 1 banana (halved or sliced) and 1/4 cup dragon fruit.

2. Into 4 small jelly jars, layer in the following order: 1/4 cup granola, 1/2 cup berries, and 2 tablespoons slivered almonds.

3. To serve, take a frozen bag of bananas and dragon fruit and transfer it to a blender. Add 1 cup of plant-based milk, and blend until smooth. Pour into a bowl. Add the contents of 1 jar of granola, berries, and almonds over the top of the smoothie, then serve with a spoon.

MANGO AND KALE SMOOTHIE

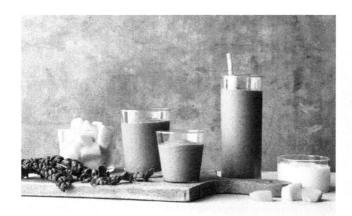

Time required:
5 minutes

Servings: 02

INGREDIENTS

2 cups oats milk, unsweetened

2 bananas, peeled

½ cup kale leaves

2 teaspoons coconut sugar

1 cup mango pieces

1 teaspoon vanilla extract, unsweetened

STEPS FOR COOKING

1. Place all the ingredients into the jar of a high-speed food processor or blender in the order stated in the ingredients list and then cover it with the lid.

2. Pulse for 1 minute until smooth, and then serve.

BAKED AVOCADO EGGS

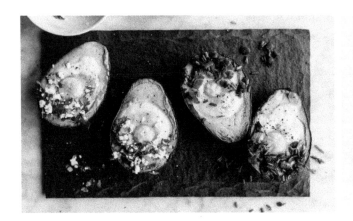

Time required:
25 minutes

Servings: 04

INGREDIENTS

*2 medium/ large
sized avocados,
halve or pitted*

4 large whole eggs

*¼ teaspoons fresh
ground black pepper*

STEPS FOR COOKING

1. Preheat your oven to 425 degrees F
2. Scoop out some pulp from the avocado halves, leaving enough space to fit an egg
3. Line an 8 by an 8-inch baking pan with foil, place avocado halves in the pan to fit nicely in a single layer
4. Gently fold the foil around the outer edges of the avocados
5. Crack 1 egg into each avocado half, season them with pepper
6. Bake for about 12-15 minutes uncovered until you have your desired doneness
7. Remove from oven, then let them rest for 5 minutes
8. Serve and enjoy!

COCONUT WATER SMOOTHIE

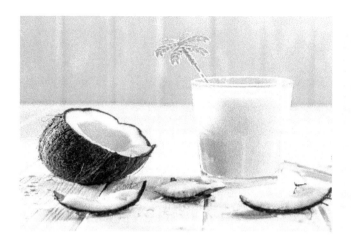

Time required:
5 minutes

Servings: 02

INGREDIENTS

2 cups of coconut water

1 large apple, peeled, cored, diced

1 cup of frozen mango pieces

2 teaspoons peanut butter

4 teaspoons coconut flakes

STEPS FOR COOKING

1. Place all the ingredients into the jar of a high-speed food processor or blender in the order stated in the ingredients list and then cover it with the lid.

2. Pulse for 1 minute until smooth, and then serve.

POTATO PANCAKES

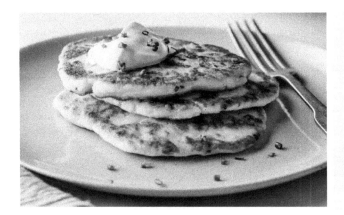

Time required:
30 minutes

Servings: 10

INGREDIENTS

½ cup white whole-wheat flour

3 large potatoes, grated

⅓ of a medium white onion, peeled, grated

1 jalapeno, minced

2 green onions, chopped

1 tablespoon minced garlic

1 teaspoon salt

¼ teaspoon baking powder

¼ teaspoon ground pepper

4 tablespoons olive oil

STEPS FOR COOKING

1. Take a large bowl, place all the ingredients except for oil and then stir until well combined; stir in 1 to 2 tablespoons water if needed to mix the batter.

2. Take a large skillet pan, place it over medium-high heat, add 2 tablespoons of oil and then let it heat.

3. Scoop the pancake mixture in portions into the pan, shape each portion like a pancake and then cook for 5 to 7 minutes per side until pancakes turn golden brown and thoroughly cooked.

4. When done, transfer the pancakes to a plate, add more oil into the pan and then cook more pancakes in the same manner.

5. Serve straight away.

BANANA AND CHIA PUDDING

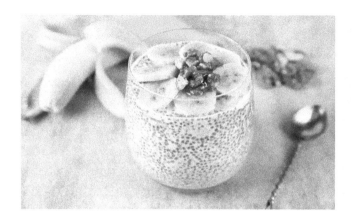

Time required:
37 minutes

Servings: 02

INGREDIENTS

For the Pudding:

2 bananas, peeled

4 tablespoons chia seeds

2 tablespoons coconut sugar

½ teaspoon pumpkin pie spice

1/8 teaspoon sea salt

½ cup almond milk, unsweetened

For the Bananas:

2 bananas, peeled, sliced

2 tablespoons coconut flakes

STEPS FOR COOKING

1. Prepare the pudding and for this, place all of its ingredients in a blender except for chia seeds and then pulse until smooth.

2. Pour the mixture into a medium saucepan, place it over medium heat, bring the mixture to a boil and then remove the pan from heat.

3. Add chia seeds into the hot banana mixture, stir until mixed, and then let it sit for 5 minutes.

4. Whisk the pudding and then let it chill for 15 minutes in the refrigerator.

5. Meanwhile, prepare the caramelized bananas and for this, take a medium skillet pan, and place it over medium heat.

6. Add banana slices, sprinkle with salt, sugar, and nutmeg, drizzle with milk

INGREDIENTS	STEPS FOR COOKING
1/8 teaspoon ground cinnamon	and then cook for 5 minutes until the mixture has thickened.
2 tablespoons coconut sugar	7. Assemble the pudding and for this, divide the pudding evenly between two bowls, top with banana slices, sprinkle with walnuts, and then serve.
¼ cup chopped walnuts	
2 tablespoons almond milk, unsweetened	

ONE-SKILLET KALE AND AVOCADO

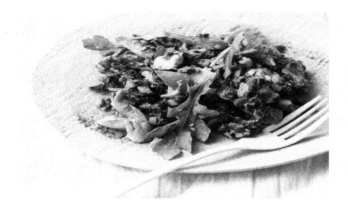

Time required:
20 minutes

Servings: 04

INGREDIENTS

2 tablespoons olive oil, divided

2 cups mushrooms, sliced

5 ounces fresh kale, stemmed and sliced into ribbons

1 avocado, sliced

4 large whole eggs

Salt and pepper as needed

STEPS FOR COOKING

1. Take a large skillet, then place it over medium heat.
2. Add a tablespoon of olive oil.
3. Add mushrooms to the pan and Saute for 3 minutes.
4. Take a medium bowl and massage kale with the remaining 1 tablespoon olive oil (for about 1-2 minutes).
5. Add kale to skillet and place them on top of mushrooms.
6. Place slices of avocado on top of the kale.
7. Create 4 wells for eggs and crack each egg onto each hold.
8. Season eggs with salt and pepper.
9. Cover skillet and cook for 5 minutes.
10. Serve hot!

HEALTHY GUACAMOLE

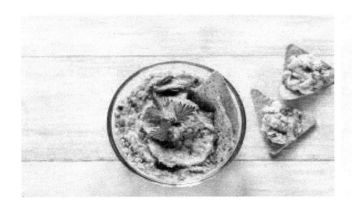

Time required:
10 minutes

Servings: 04

INGREDIENTS

3 large ripe avocados

1 large red onion, peeled and diced

4 tablespoon of freshly squeezed lime juice

Salt as needed

Freshly ground black pepper as needed

Cayenne pepper as needed

STEPS FOR COOKING

1. Halve the avocados and discard the stone.
2. Scoop flesh from 3 avocado halves and transfer to a large bowl.
3. Mash using a fork.
4. Add 2 tablespoon of lime juice and mix.
5. Dice the remaining avocado flesh (remaining half) and transfer to another bowl.
6. Add remaining juice and toss.
7. Add diced flesh with the mashed flesh and mix.
8. Add chopped onions and toss.
9. Season with salt, pepper, and cayenne pepper.
10. Serve and enjoy!

GRILLED ZUCCHINI MEAL

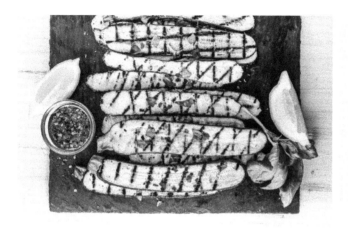

Time required:
70 minutes

Servings: 04

INGREDIENTS

Olive oil as needed

3 zucchinis

½ teaspoon black pepper

½ teaspoon mustard

½ teaspoon cumin

1 teaspoon paprika

1 teaspoon garlic powder

1 tablespoon of sea salt

1-2 stevia

1 tablespoon chili powder

STEPS FOR COOKING

1. Preheat your oven to 300 degrees F.

2. Take a small bowl. Add cayenne, black pepper, salt, garlic, mustard, paprika, chili powder, and stevia, then mix well.

3. Slice zucchini into 1/8 inch slices and mist them with olive oil.

4. Sprinkle spice blend over Zucchini and bake for 40 minutes.

5. Remove and flip, mist with more olive oil and leftover spice.

6. Bake for 20 minutes more.

7. Serve!

TANGY BROCCOLI SALAD

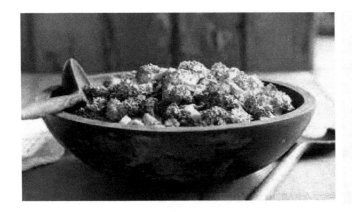

Time required:
15 minutes

Servings: 04

INGREDIENTS

2 heads broccoli, stems, and florets chopped (about 5 cups)

3 scallions, thinly sliced

½ cup carrots, grated

¼ cup hemp hearts

2 tablespoons tahini

2 tablespoons apple cider vinegar

2 tablespoons water

2 teaspoons maple syrup

1 garlic clove

¼ teaspoon salt

Freshly ground black pepper

STEPS FOR COOKING

1. Place the broccoli, scallions, carrots, and hemp hearts in a large bowl. Whisk the tahini, vinegar, water, maple syrup, garlic, and salt in a measuring cup or small bowl. Add pepper to taste.

2. Put the dressing over the salad and mix until everything is well combined.

RICE ARUGULA SALAD

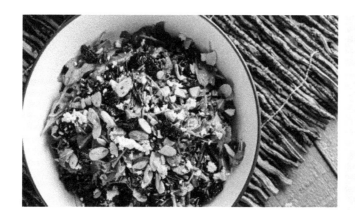

Time required:
23 minutes

Servings: 02

1 cup wild rice, cooked

1 handful arugula, washed

¾ cup almonds

6 sun-dried tomatoes in oil, chopped

3 tablespoons olive oil

1 onion

Pepper and salt, to taste

1. Put your frying pan over low heat and roast the almonds for 3 minutes. Transfer to a salad bowl.

2. Sauté onions in 1/3 olive oil for 3 minutes on low heat. Add dried tomatoes and cook for about 2 minutes. Transfer to a bowl.

3. Add the remaining olive oil to the pan and fry the bread until crunchy. Sprinkle with pepper and salt. Set aside.

4. Place arugula into the bowl containing sautéed tomato mixture, then add the wild rice and toss to combine. Season with pepper, salt.

SWEET POTATO HASH AND FRIED EGGS

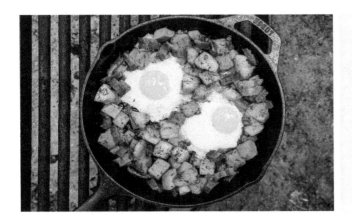

Time required:
25 minutes

Servings: 02

INGREDIENTS

For the hash:

1 large garnet yam

1 big pinch of kosher salt

For the eggs:

Several turns of freshly ground black pepper

A few shakes of garlic powder

A couple of dashes of onion powder

A sprinkle of dried herbs

2 tablespoons fat

4 large eggs

1 tablespoon ghee or avocado oil

STEPS FOR COOKING

1. Grab a yam or seven, depending on how many folks you'll be feeding.

2. Peel and cut the yam lengthwise so the slices fit in the feeding tube of your food processor. Attach the julienne slicer blade to the machine and shred the yams. (Alternatively, you can use a spiralizer to make sweet potato "noodles.")

3. Transfer the shredded yams to a large bowl and toss with salt, pepper, garlic and onion powders, and dried herbs. You can definitely substitute fresh alliums and herbs if you've got them. Taste the mixture and adjust the seasoning.

4. Heat the fat in a large cast iron skillet over medium heat. When the oil is

Kosher salt

Freshly ground black pepper A

leppo pepper

optional

shimmering, add the seasoned sweet potatoes/yams.

5. Toss everything in the fat and stir-fry for a minute. Then, pop on a lid for a few more minutes while the yams cook. The hash is ready when there's some crunchy brown bits and texture is soft and tender.

6. You can plate it up with a dash of Aleppo pepper and gobble up the hash by itself or you can split the hash into two servings and top each dish with a couple of sunny-side-up eggs. The addition of the eggs brings a wonderful richness to the hash, making this a full and well-rounded dish with plenty o' fat and protein to go with the carbs.

7. Add a tablespoon of ghee to a hot 8-inch cast iron skillet over medium-low heat. When the fat shimmers, crack two eggs into a bowl and pour 'em gently into the hot pan.

8. Season the eggs with salt and pepper, and cover with a lid for 2-3 minutes, depending on how runny you like your yolks.

9. Once they're done, carefully slide them out of the skillet and on top of a mound of hash. Repeat with the remaining eggs. Sprinkle some more Aleppo pepper on top.

SCALLION AND MINT SOUP

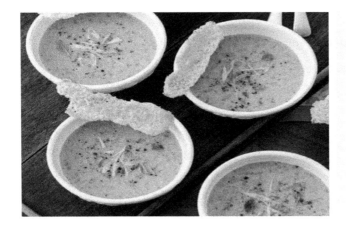

Time required:
20 minutes

Servings: 04

INGREDIENTS

6 cups vegetable broth

¼ cup fresh mint leaves, roughly chopped

¼ cup chopped scallions (the white and green parts)

3 garlic cloves, minced

3 tablespoons freshly squeezed lime juice

STEPS FOR COOKING

1. In a large stockpot, mix the broth, mint, scallions, garlic, and lime juice, then bring to a boil over medium-high heat.

2. Reduce the heat to low, cover, then simmer for 15 minutes, and serve.

CHICKEN AND BASIL ZUCCHINI ZOODLES

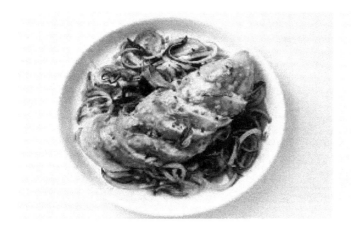

Time required:
20 minutes

Servings: 04

INGREDIENTS

2 chicken fillets, cubed

2 tablespoons ghee

1 pound tomatoes, diced

½ cup basil, chopped

¼ cup of coconut milk

1 garlic clove, peeled, minced

1 zucchini, shredded

STEPS FOR COOKING

1. Sauté cubed chicken in ghee until no longer pink
2. Add tomatoes and season with salt
3. Simmer and reduce the liquid
4. Prepare your zucchini Zoodles by shredding zucchini in a food processor
5. Add basil, garlic, coconut milk to chicken and cook for a few minutes
6. Add half of the zucchini Zoodles to a bowl and top with creamy tomato basil chicken
7. Enjoy!

PARSLEY CHICKEN BREAST

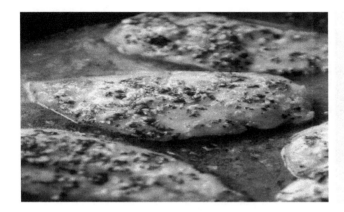

Time required:
50 minutes

Servings: 04

INGREDIENTS

1 tablespoon dry parsley

1 tablespoon dry basil

4 chicken breast halves, boneless and skinless

½ teaspoon salt

½ teaspoon red pepper flakes, crushed

2 tomatoes, sliced

STEPS FOR COOKING

1. Preheat your oven to 350 degrees F.
2. Take a 9x13 inch baking dish and grease it up with cooking spray.
3. Sprinkle 1 tablespoon of parsley, 1 teaspoon of basil, and spread the mixture over your baking dish.
4. Arrange the chicken breast halves over the dish, then sprinkle garlic slices on top.
5. Take a small bowl and add 1 teaspoon parsley, 1 teaspoon of basil, salt, basil, red pepper, and mix well. Pour over the chicken breast.
6. Top with tomato slices and cover, bake for 25 minutes.
7. Remove the cover and bake for 15 minutes.
8. Serve and enjoy!

ALMOND AND TOMATO SALAD

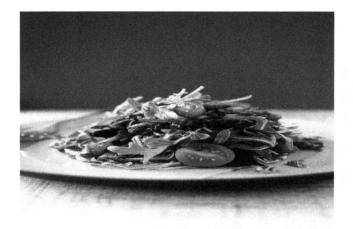

Time required:
25 minutes

Servings: 04

INGREDIENTS

1 medium zucchini

1 tablespoon grated red onion

2 extra-large eggs lightly beaten

3 tablespoons all-purpose flour

½ tablespoons ground black pepper

½ tablespoon salt

vegetable oil

1 teaspoon of baking powder

STEPS FOR COOKING

1. Preheat the oven to over 300 degrees Fahrenheit.

2. In a mixing bowl, grate the zucchini and add the onions and eggs right away.

3. Combine the flour, baking powder, salt, and pepper in a mixing bowl.

4. Add the vegetable oil to a big sauté pan and steam over medium heat.

5. Reduce the heat to medium-low and pour the batter into the pan once the oil is hot. Cook both sides for about 2 minutes.

FIG AND KALE SALAD

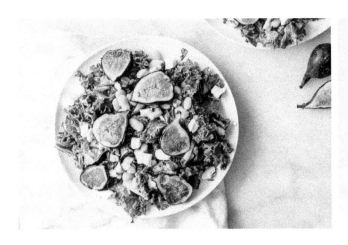

Time required:
15 minutes

Servings: 02

INGREDIENTS

1 ripe avocado

2 tablespoons lemon juice

3 ½ oz kale, packed, stems removed and cut into large-sized bits

1 carrot, shredded

1 yellow zucchini, diced

4 fresh figs

¼ cup ground flaxseed

1 cup mixed green leaves

1 teaspoon sea saltr

STEPS FOR COOKING

1. Add kale to a bowl with avocado, lemon juice, and sea salt. Massage together until kale wilts.

2. Add in zucchini, carrot, and 2 cups mixed green leaves. Fold in figs and remaining ingredients.

3. Toss and serve.

PESTO AND WHITE BEAN PASTA SALAD

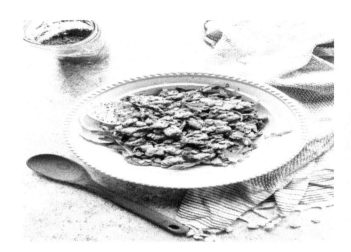

Time required:
25 minutes

Servings: 04

INGREDIENTS

1.1/2 cups canned cannellini beans

1/2 cup Spinach Pesto

1 cup chopped tomato or red bell pepper

1/4 red onion, finely diced

1/2 cup chopped pitted black olives

STEPS FOR COOKING

1. In a large bowl, place pasta, beans, and pesto, then toss to combine.

2. Add the tomato, red onion, and olives. Toss and serve.

STEAMED MUSSELS IN WHITE WINE SAUCE

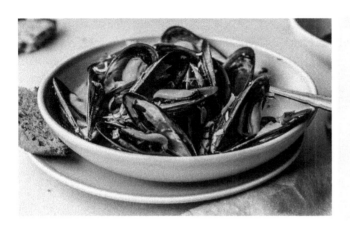

Time required:
15 minutes

Servings: 04

INGREDIENTS

2 pounds small mussels

1 tablespoon extra virgin olive oil

1 cup sliced red onion

3 garlic cloves, sliced

1 cup dry white wine

2 (1/4-inch-thick) lemon slices

1/4 teaspoon freshly ground black pepper

1/4 teaspoon kosher or sea salt

Fresh lemon wedges, for serving (optional)

STEPS FOR COOKING

1. In a large colander in the sink, run cold water over the mussels (but don't let the mussels sit in standing water). All the shells should be closed tight; discard any shells that are a little bit open or any shells that are cracked. Leave the mussels in the colander until you're ready to use them.

2. Heat the oil in a skillet. Attach the onion and cook,

3. Add the mussels and cover. Cook in low heat.

4. All the shells should now be wide open. Using a slotted spoon, discard any mussels that are still closed. Spoon the opened mussels into a shallow serving bowl, and pour the

broth over the top. Serve with
additional fresh lemon slices, if
desired.

ROASTED SHRIMP-GNOCCHI BAKE

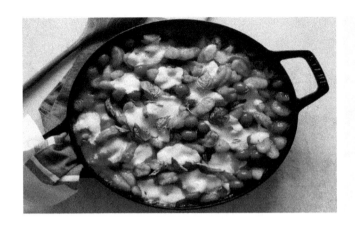

Time required:
30 minutes

Servings: 06

1 cup tomato

2 tablespoons extra-virgin olive oil

2 garlic cloves, minced

1/2 teaspoon black pepper

1/4 teaspoon crushed red pepper

1 jarred peppers

1-pound fresh raw shrimp

1-pound frozen gnocchi

1/2 cup cubed feta cheese

1/3 cup fresh torn basil leaves

1. Preheat the oven to 425°F.

2. In a baking dish, mix the tomatoes, oil, garlic, black pepper, and crushed red pepper, then roast in the oven for 10 minutes.

3. Stir in the roasted peppers and shrimp, then roast for 10 more minutes, until the shrimp turn pink and white.

4. While the shrimp cooks, cook the gnocchi on the stovetop according to the package directions. Drain in a colander, then keep warm.

5. Remove the dish from the oven. Mix in the cooked gnocchi, feta, and basil, and serve.

PESTO PASTA

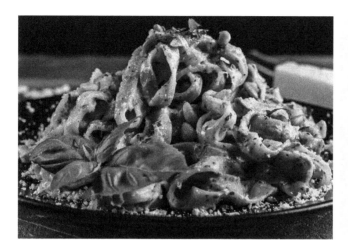

Time required:
18 minutes

Servings: 02

INGREDIENTS

1 cup fresh basil leaves

4 cloves garlic

2 tablespoons walnut

2 tablespoons olive oil

1 tablespoon vegan Parmesan cheese

2 cups cooked penne pasta

2 tablespoons black olives, sliced

STEPS FOR COOKING

1. Put the basil leaves, garlic, walnut, olive oil, and Parmesan cheese in a food processor.
2. Pulse until smooth.
3. Divide pasta into 2 food containers.
4. Spread the basil sauce on top.
5. Top with black olives.
6. Store until ready to serve.

VEGAN TACOS

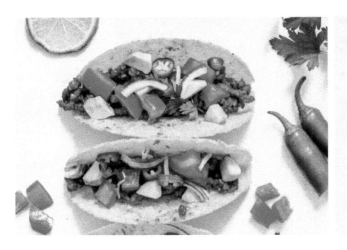

Time required:
30 minutes

Servings: 04

INGREDIENTS

1/2 teaspoon onion powder

1/2 teaspoon garlic powder

1 teaspoon chili powder

2 tablespoons tamari

16 oz. tofu drained and crumbled

1 tablespoon olive oil

1 ripe avocado

1 tablespoon vegan mayonnaise

1 teaspoon lime juice

STEPS FOR COOKING

1. Merge all the ingredients in a bowl.
2. Marinate the tofu in this mixture for about 10 mins.
3. Pour the oil into a pan over medium heat, then cook the tofu mixture for 10 minutes.
4. In another bowl, mash the avocado and mix with mayo, lime juice, and salt.
5. Stuff each corn tortilla with tofu mixture, mashed avocado, salsa, and lettuce.
6. Serve with pickled radishes.

Salt to taste

8 corn tortillas, warmed

1/2 cup fresh salsa

2 cups iceberg lettuce, shredded

Pickled radishes

BAKED HALIBUT DELIGHT

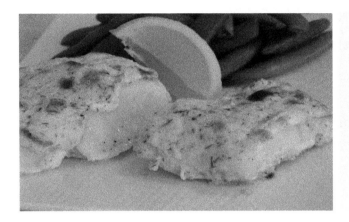

Time required:
40 minutes

Servings: 04

INGREDIENTS

6 ounces halibut
fillets

1 tablespoon Greek
seasoning

1 large tomato,
chopped

1 onion, chopped

5 ounces kalamata
olives, pitted

¼ cup capers

¼ cup olive oil

1 tablespoon lemon
juice

Salt and pepper as
needed

STEPS FOR COOKING

1. Preheat your oven to 350 degrees
   Fahrenheit.

2. Transfer the halibut fillets on a large
   aluminum foil.

3. Season with Greek seasoning.

4. Take a bowl and add tomato, onion,
   olives, olive oil, capers, pepper, lemon
   juice, and salt.

5. Mix well and spoon the tomato mix
   over the halibut.

6. Seal the edges and fold to make a
   packet.

7. Place the packet on a baking sheet
   and bake in your oven for 30-40
   minutes.

8. Serve once the fish flakes off, and
   enjoy!

9. Serve over rice cauliflower if desired.

CABBAGE FRIED BEEF MEAL

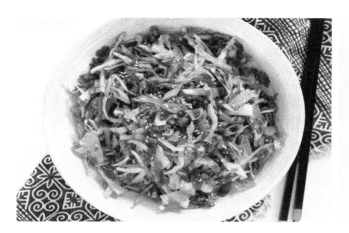

Time required:
25 minutes

Servings: 04

INGREDIENTS

STEPS FOR COOKING

1 pound beef, ground

½ pound bacon

1 onion

1 garlic cloves, minced

½ head cabbage, sliced

Salt, and pepper to taste

1. Take a skillet, then place it over medium heat.

2. Add chopped bacon, beef, and onion until slightly browned.

3. Transfer to a bowl and keep it covered.

4. Add minced garlic and cabbage to the skillet and cook until slightly browned.

5. Return the ground beef mixture to the skillet and simmer for 3-5 minutes over low heat.

6. Serve and enjoy!

PUMPKIN SPICY CHILI DELIGHT

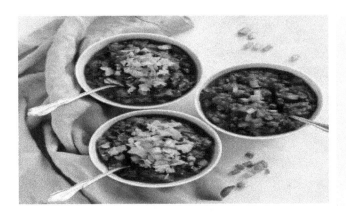

Time required:
25 minutes

Servings: 04

INGREDIENTS

3 cups yellow onion, chopped

8 garlic cloves, chopped

1 pound turkey, ground

2 cans (15 ounces each) fire-roasted tomatoes

2 cups pumpkin puree

1 cup chicken broth

4 teaspoons chili spice

1 teaspoon ground cinnamon

1 teaspoon of sea salt

STEPS FOR COOKING

1. Take a large-sized pot, then place it over medium-high heat.

2. Add coconut oil and let the oil heat up.

3. Add onion and garlic, then Sauté for 5 minutes.

4. Add ground turkey and break it while cooking; cook for 5 minutes.

5. Add remaining ingredients and bring the mix to simmer.

6. Simmer for 15 minutes over low heat (lid off).

7. Pour chicken broth.

8. Serve with desired salad.

9. Enjoy!

SPLIT PEA SOUP

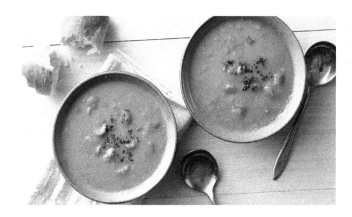

Time required:
75 minutes

Servings: 06

2 tablespoons olive oil

1 medium onion, coarsely chopped

2 carrots, coarsely chopped

2 celery stalks, coarsely chopped

Pinch + 2 teaspoons salt, divided

2 cups yellow split peas, drained

8 cups of water

1 bay leaf

1 teaspoon paprika

Freshly ground black pepper

6 cups spinach, chopped

1. In a large stockpot, warm the oil over medium heat, then add the onion, carrots, celery, and a pinch of salt and cook until the onions start to soften.

2. Add the split peas, water, bay leaf, paprika, remaining 2 teaspoons of salt, and pepper. Bring to a boil.

3. Adjust the heat to low, then simmer, occasionally stirring, until the split peas are soft and the soup is thick about 50 minutes.

4. Remove and discard the bay leaf. Stir in the spinach and sausage (if using) and cook for a couple of minutes more—taste, adjust seasonings with salt and pepper.

INGREDIENTS

STEPS FOR COOKING

2 vegan sausages or spicy store-bought, chopped (optional)

ROASTED PINE NUT ORZO

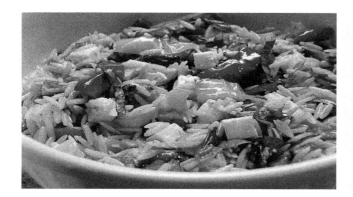

Time required:
25 minutes

Servings: 03

16 ounces orzo

1 cup diced roasted red peppers

1/4 cup pitted, chopped Klamath olives

4 garlic cloves, minced or pressed

3 tablespoons olive oil

1.1/2 tablespoons squeezed lemon juice

2 teaspoons balsamic vinegar

1 teaspoon sea salt

1/4 cup pine nuts

1/4 cup packed thinly sliced or torn fresh basil

1. Use a large pot of water to a boil over medium-high heat and add the orzo. Cook, stirring often, for 10 minutes, or until the orzo has a chewy and firm texture. Drain well.

2. While the orzo is cooking, in a large bowl, combine the peppers, olives, garlic, olive oil, lemon juice, vinegar, and salt. Stir well.

3. In a dry skillet toasts the pine nuts over medium-low heat until aromatic and lightly browned, shaking the pan often so that they cook evenly.

4. Upon reaching the desired texture and add it to the sauce mixture within a minute or so, to avoid clumping.

BEEF STROGANOFF

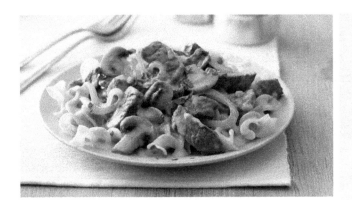

Time required:
4 hours

Servings: 02

INGREDIENTS

1/2 lb. beef stew
meat

10 oz mushroom
soup, homemade

1 medium onion,
chopped

1/2 cup sour cream

oz mushrooms,
sliced

Pepper, and salt

STEPS FOR COOKING

1. Add all the ingredients excluding sour
   cream into a pot and mix well.

2. Cover and cook on low flame for 4
   hours.

3. Add sour cream and stir well.

4. Serve and enjoy.

LEMON LAMB LEG

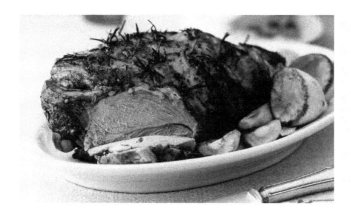

Time required:
2 hours

Servings: 08

INGREDIENTS

4 lbs. lamb leg, boneless and a slice of fat

1 tablespoon rosemary, crushed

1/4 cup water

1/4 cup lemon juice

1 teaspoon black pepper

1/4 teaspoon salt

STEPS FOR COOKING

1. Place lamb into a pot.
2. Add remaining ingredients over the lamb, into the pot.
3. Cover then cook on low flame for 2 hours.
4. Remove lamb from the pot and slice it.
5. Serve and enjoy.

Mushroom Pork Chops

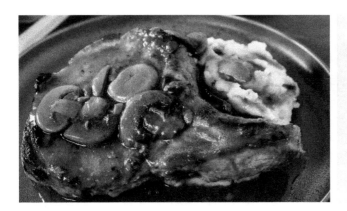

Time required:
50 minutes

Servings: 04

INGREDIENTS

8 ounces
mushrooms, sliced

1 teaspoon garlic

1 onion, peeled and
chopped

1 cup Keto-Friendly
Mayonnaise

3 pork chops,
boneless

1 teaspoon ground
nutmeg

1 tablespoon
balsamic vinegar

½ cup of coconut oil

STEPS FOR COOKING

1. Place a pan over medium heat.
2. Add oil and let it heat up.
3. Add mushrooms, onions, and stir.
4. Cook for 4 minutes, then add pork chops, season with nutmeg, garlic powder, and brown both sides.
5. Transfer the pan to the oven and bake for 30 minutes at 350 degrees F.
6. Transfer pork chops to plates and keep them warm.
7. Take a pan and place it over medium heat.
8. Add vinegar, mayonnaise over the mushroom mixture and stir for a few minutes.
9. Drizzle sauce over pork chops.
10. Enjoy!

ONION THYME CRACKER

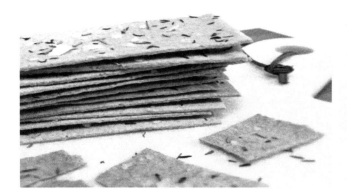

Time required:
130 minutes

Servings: 75

INGREDIENTS

1 garlic clove, minced

1 cup sweet onion, coarsely chopped

2 teaspoon fresh thyme leaves

¼ cup avocado oil

¼ teaspoon Himalayan salt

Freshly ground black pepper

¼ cup sunflower seeds

1 and ½ cups roughly ground flax seeds

STEPS FOR COOKING

1. Preheat your oven to 225 degrees F.
2. Line two baking sheets with parchment paper and keep it on the side.
3. Place garlic, onion, thyme, oil, salt, and pepper into a food processor.
4. Add sunflower and flax seeds, pulse until pureed, then transfer batter to prepared baking sheets and spread evenly, cut into crackers.
5. Bake for 60 minutes.
6. Remove parchment paper and flip crackers, bake for another hour.
7. Remove from oven and let them cool.
8. Enjoy!

TOFU SCRAMBLE

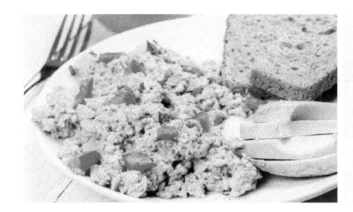

Time required:
20 minutes

Servings: 03

INGREDIENTS

12 ounces tofu, extra-firm, pressed, drained

½ of a medium red onion, peeled, sliced

1 cup baby greens mix

1 medium red bell pepper, cored, sliced

½ teaspoon garlic powder

1 teaspoon salt

½ teaspoon ground black pepper

¼ teaspoon turmeric powder

¼ teaspoon ground cumin

STEPS FOR COOKING

1. Take a large bowl, place tofu in it, and then break it into bite-size pieces.

2. Add salt, black pepper, turmeric, and 2 tablespoons of oil, and then stir until mixed.

3. Take a medium skillet pan, place it over medium heat, add garlic powder and cumin and then cook for 1 minute until fragrant.

4. Add tofu mixture, stir until mixed, switch heat to medium-high level, and then cook for 5 minutes until tofu turn golden brown.

5. When done, divide tofu evenly between three plates, keep it warm, and then set aside until required.

6. Return the skillet pan over medium-high heat, add remaining oil and let it heat until hot.

INGREDIENTS	STEPS FOR COOKING

4 tablespoons olive oil, divided

7. Add onion and bell peppers, cook for 5 to 7 minutes or until beginning to brown, and then season with a pinch of salt.

8. Add baby greens, toss until mixed, and then cook for 30 seconds until leaves begin to wilts.

9. Add vegetables evenly to the plates to scrambled tofu and then serve.

CHICKPEA FLOUR FRITTATA

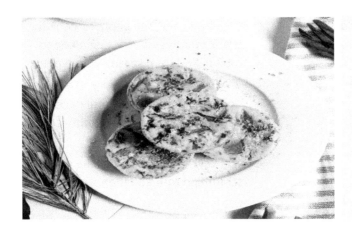

Time required:
60 minutes

Servings: 06

INGREDIENTS

STEPS FOR COOKING

*1 medium green bell
pepper, cored,
chopped*

*1 cup chopped
greens*

*1 cup cauliflower
florets, chopped*

*½ cup chopped
broccoli florets*

*½ of a medium red
onion, peeled and
chopped*

¼ teaspoon salt

*½ cup chopped
zucchini*

For the Batter:

¼ cup cashew cream

½ cup chickpea flour

1. Switch on the oven, then set it to 375
   degrees F, then let it preheat.
2. Take a 9-inch pie pan, grease it with
   oil, and then set aside until required.
3. Take a large bowl, place all the
   vegetables in it, sprinkle with salt and
   then toss until combined.
4. Prepare the batter and for this, add all
   of its ingredients in it except for
   thyme, dill, and cilantro and then
   pulse until combined and smooth.
5. Pour the batter over the vegetables,
   add dill, thyme, and cilantro, and then
   stir until combined.
6. Spoon the mixture into the prepared
   pan, spread evenly, and then bake for
   45 to 50 minutes until done and

INGREDIENTS	STEPS FOR COOKING
½ cup chopped cilantro *½ teaspoon salt* *¼ teaspoon cayenne pepper* *½ teaspoon dried dill* *¼ teaspoon ground black pepper* *¼ teaspoon dried thyme* *½ teaspoon ground turmeric* *1 tablespoon olive oil* *1 ½ cup water*	inserted toothpick into frittata comes out clean. 7. When done, let the frittata rest for 10 minutes, cut it into slices, and then serve.

Easy Summer Gazpacho

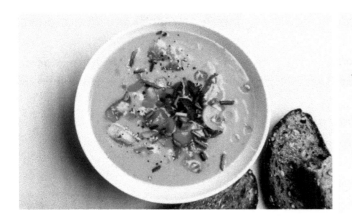

Time required:
15 minutes

Servings: 02

INGREDIENTS

STEPS FOR COOKING

1.5 lbs. ripe tomatoes on the vine, cut into 1/2 inch wedges and seeds removed

1/2 hothouse cucumber, peeled and seeded (about 1.5 cups diced large)

1 stalk of celery, cut into 1 inch chunks

1 small red bell pepper, seeds/core removed and cut into 1 inch chunks

1 medium shallot, diced

1 clove garlic

1. In a high powered blender (I use my Vitamix), combine the tomatoes, cucumbers, red bell pepper, celery, shallot, garlic, olive oil, kosher salt, black pepper, and the balsamic vinegar. Blend on high until smooth.

2. Serve in bowls and garnish with halved cherry tomatoes, diced cucumber, a drizzle of extra virgin olive oil, a sprinkle of kosher salt and freshly cracked black pepper, and freshly chopped chives-- if desired. Enjoy!

1/4 cup extra virgin olive oil (plus more for serving)

1 teaspoon kosher salt

2 tablespoons balsamic vinegar

diced cucumber, for serving (if desired)

halved cherry tomatoes, for serving (if desired)

GARDEN EGG SALAD

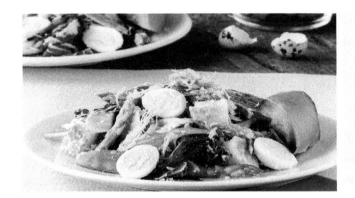

Time required:
35 minutes

Servings: 04

INGREDIENTS

6 large eggs

½ cup low-fat mayonnaise

2 Tbsp whole-grain mustard

Kosher salt and freshly ground black pepper

2 scallions (white and green), thinly sliced

1 rib celery, minced, scant 1/2 cup

2 radishes, grated on the large holes of a box grater

8 Romaine lettuce leaves

1 cup pea or other sprouts

STEPS FOR COOKING

1. Put the eggs in a saucepan with enough cold water to cover. Bring to a boil, cover, and remove from the heat. Set aside for 12 minutes. Drain the eggs and roll them between your palm and the counter to crack the shell, then peel under cool running water.

2. Dice the eggs. Combine the eggs with mayonnaise, mustard and season with the salt and pepper. Stir in the scallions, celery, and radish.

3. Divide the egg salad among the lettuce leaves, top with the sprouts and roll up. Serve 2 rolls per serving.

HUMMUS AND OLIVE PITA BREAD

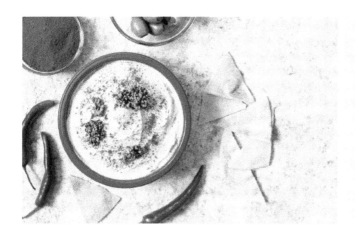

Time required:
5 minutes

Servings: 03

INGREDIENTS

7 pita bread cut into 6 wedges each

1 (7 ounces) container plain hummus

1 tbsp Greek vinaigrette

½ cup Chopped pitted Kalamata olives

STEPS FOR COOKING

1. Spread the hummus on a serving plate. Mix vinaigrette and olives in a bowl and spoon over the hummus.

2. Enjoy with wedges of pita bread.

HEARTY TOMATO SALAD

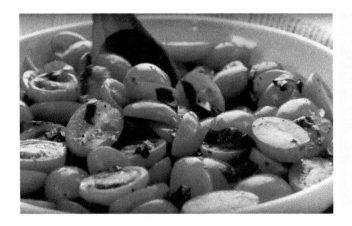

Time required:
35 minutes

Servings: 04

INGREDIENTS

½ cup scallions,
chopped

1 pound cherry
tomatoes

3 teaspoons olive oil

Sea salt and ground
black pepper

1 tablespoon red
wine vinegar

STEPS FOR COOKING

1. Season tomatoes with spices and oil
2. Heat your oven to 450 degrees Fahrenheit
3. Take a baking sheet, then spread the tomatoes
4. Bake for 15 minutes
5. Stir and turn the tomatoes
6. Then again, bake for 10 minutes
7. Take a bowl and mix the roasted tomatoes with all the remaining ingredients
8. Serve and enjoy!

PUMPKIN AND BRUSSELS SPROUTS MIX

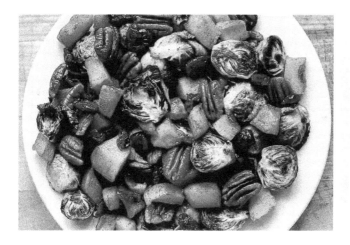

Time required:
65 minutes

Servings: 08

INGREDIENTS

1 lb. Brussels sprouts halved

1 pumpkin, peeled, cubed

4 garlic cloves, sliced

2 tablespoons fresh parsley, chopped

2 tablespoons balsamic vinegar

1/3 cup olive oil

Salt, pepper, to taste

STEPS FOR COOKING

1. Warm oven to 400 degrees F. Prepare a baking dish and coat with cooking spray. Mix sprouts, pumpkin, and garlic in a bowl, then add oil and toss well to coat the vegetables.

2. Transfer to the baking dish and cook for 35-40 minutes. Stir once halfway. Serve topped with parsley.

VEGAN PALEO BROWNIES

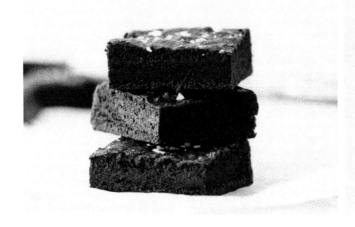

Time required:
70 minutes

Servings: 08

INGREDIENTS

1½ cups boiled black
(Beluga) lentils

25g nut or seed
butter (without
additives)

200g of oat milk

4 tbsps. coconut
flour

1 tbsp. mesquite
flour

2 tbsps. carob
powder

2 tbsps. cocoa
powder

1 tsp. cinnamon

1½ tsp. psyllium
powder

STEPS FOR COOKING

1. Start with soaking Beluga lentils for 8 hours. Then rinse, drain and boil the lentils. 2 cups of boiled lentils is about 115g (4.06oz) dry lentils. Or buy enough of canned lentils. Make sure to rinse and drain those as well.

2. Next, add all the ingredients (except chocolate chips and cocoa nibs) into food processor and process until you have homogeneous and smooth batter. You'll need to scrape the sides every now and then.

3. Then, transfer the batter onto baking sheet lined with parchment paper and spread it out into about 17x17cm (6.8 inch) square.

4. Finally, sprinkle on some chocolate chips and cocoa nibs, press them

3 tbsps. birch xylitol or stevia to taste

¼ tsp. Himalayan salt

2 tsps. dark chocolate chips

1 tsp. cocoa nibs

down and bake the brownies at 175°C (350°F) for 35 minutes. Let cool before slicing.

ALMOND BUTTER ICEBOX PIE

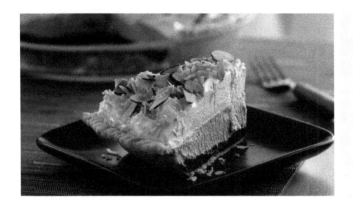

Time required:
60 minutes

Servings: 04

INGREDIENTS

STEPS FOR COOKING

Almond Crust:

1 1/2 cups almonds

3 Tbs coconut oil

generous pinch pink salt

1 tsp vanilla extract

Vanilla Almond Cream:

3/4 cup natural almond butter

1 13.7 oz can coconut milk, solid cream only - 3/4 cup

3 Tbs light amber maple syrup - or 25-35 drops stevia or monkfruit +3 T coconut milk for keto

To make the crust:

1. Add almonds to a food processor. Pulse a few times to break down. Add oil, salt and vanilla and pulse until finely ground.

2. Scoop 1 heaping Tbs to 10 silicone molds or foil cupcake wrappers (I used a cookie scoop) and press firmly. Chill crusts in the fridge while you prepare the filling.

To make the cream filling:

1. (Use a can of coconut milk that has been refrigerated for a minimum of 24 hours.) Scoop out the solid cream into a mixing bowl. If your cream is too hard, whip with a hand mixer first. Add remaining ingredients (except garnish) and whisk smooth. Taste and adjust for sweetness.

2 Tbs vanilla extract

pinch pink salt

dark chocolate, sliced almonds and cacao nibs - for garnish (use Lily's sugar-free chocolate for keto)

2. Top each crust with a scoop of cream filling. (I used an ice cream scoop) Tap tray on the counter several times and stir each pie to release air bubbles.

3. Freeze for about 2 hours to set. Garnish with melted chocolate, cacao nibs and almond slivers if you like.

4. Thaw on the counter for about 10 minutes to soften slightly. ENJOY!

VEGAN EXOTIC CHOCOLATE MOUSSE

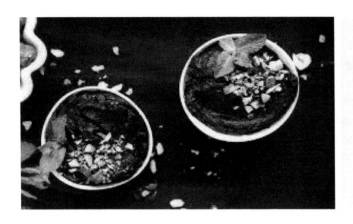

Time required:
10 minutes

Servings: 04

INGREDIENTS

2 frozen bananas chunk

2 avocados

1/3 cup of dates

4 Tbsp. cocoa powder

1/2 cup of fresh orange juice

Zest, from 1 orange

STEPS FOR COOKING

1. Add bananas, avocado, and dates to a food processor.

2. Process for about 2 to 3 minutes until combined well.

3. Add cocoa powder, orange juice, and orange zest; process for a further one minute.

4. Place cream in a glass jar or container and keep refrigerated for up to one week.

SEASONED CINNAMON MANGO POPSICLES

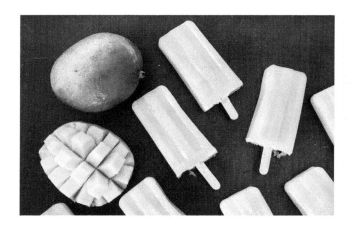

Time required:
15 minutes

Servings: 06

INGREDIENTS

1 1/2 cups of mango pulp

1 mango cut in cubes

1 cup brown sugar (packed)

2 Tbsp. lemon juice freshly squeezed

1 tsp. cinnamon

1 pinch of salt

STEPS FOR COOKING

1. Add all ingredients to your blender.
2. Blend until brown sugar dissolved.
3. Pour the mango mixture evenly in Popsicle molds or cups.
4. Insert sticks into each mold.
5. Place molds in a freezer, and freeze for at least 5 to6 hours.
6. Before serving, un-mold easy your popsicles placing molds under lukewarm water.

FETA CHEESECAKE

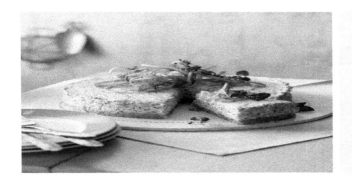

Time required:
120 minutes

Servings: 12

INGREDIENTS

2 cups graham
cracker crumbs
(about 30 crackers)

½ tsp ground
cinnamon

6 tbsps. Unsalted
butter, melted

½ cup sesame seeds,
toasted

12 ounces cream
cheese, softened

1 cup crumbled feta
cheese

1 cup of sugar

2 cups plain yogurt

2 tbsps. Grated
lemon zest

1 tsp vanilla

STEPS FOR COOKING

1. Set the oven to 350° F.

2. Mix the cracker crumbs, butter,
   cinnamon, and sesame seeds with a
   fork. Move the combination to a
   springform pan and spread until it is
   even. Refrigerate.

3. In a separate bowl, mix the cream
   cheese and feta. With an electric
   mixer, beat both kinds of cheese
   together., beating the mixture with
   each new addition. Add sugar, then
   keep beating until creamy. Mix in
   yogurt, vanilla, and lemon zest.

4. Bring out the refrigerated springform
   and spread the batter on it. Then
   place it in a baking pan. Pour water
   into the pan till it is halfway full.

5. Bake for about 50 minutes. Remove
   cheesecake and allow it to cool.
   Refrigerate for at least 4 hours.

6. It is done. Serve when ready.

VANILLA CUPCAKES

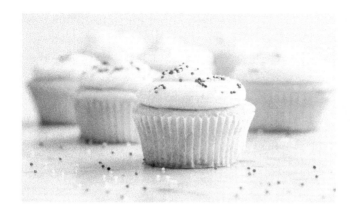

Time required:
30 minutes

Servings: 18

INGREDIENTS

STEPS FOR COOKING

2 cups white whole-wheat flour

1 cup of coconut sugar

½ teaspoon salt

2 teaspoons baking powder

1 ¼ teaspoons vanilla extract, unsweetened

½ teaspoon baking soda

1 tablespoon apple cider vinegar

½ cup coconut oil, melted

1 ½ cups almond milk, unsweetened

1. Set the oven to 350 degrees F, and then let it preheat.

2. Meanwhile, take a medium bowl, place vinegar in it, stir in milk, and then let it stand for 5 minutes until curdled.

3. Take a large bowl, place flour in it, add salt, baking soda and powder, and sugar and then stir until mixed.

4. Take a separate large bowl, pour in curdled milk mixture, add vanilla and coconut oil and then whisk until combined.

5. Whisk almond milk mixture into the flour mixture until smooth batter comes together, and then spoon the mixture into two 12- cups muffin pans lined with muffin cups.

6. Bake the muffins for 15 to 20 minutes until firm and the top turn golden brown, and then let them cool on the wire rack completely.

7. Serve straight away.

Lightning Source UK Ltd.
Milton Keynes UK
UKHW050320110521
383304UK00004B/14